GOD'S
MEDICINE
IS BEST

GOD'S MEDICINE IS BEST

HERBS, VITAMINS AND MINERALS

LINDA WISE

To order additional copies of this book, contact:
Xlibris Corporation
1-888-795-4274
www.Xlibris.com
Orders@Xlibris.com
41796

CONTENTS

E

F

G

H

I

J

K

L

M

N

O

P

R

S

T

U

V

W

X

I WOULD LIKE TO THANK MY HUSBAND

AND MY CHILDREN FOR THEIR TREMENDOUS SUPPORT

IN WRITING THIS BOOK.

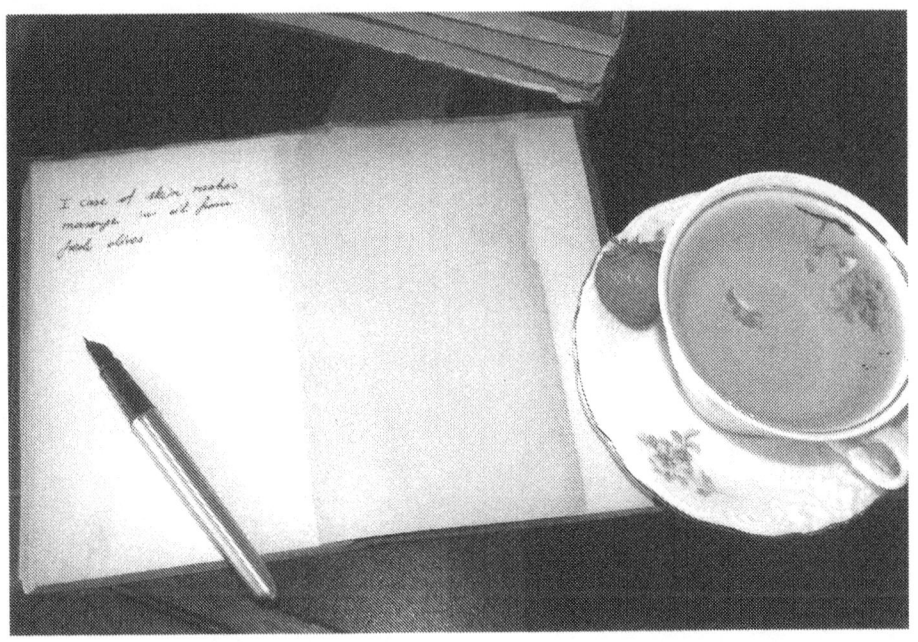

TO THE MEMORY OF MY GRANDMOTHER, JANINA S.

WHO DIED RIGHT AFTER THE WORLD WAR II.

INTRODUCTION

THIS BOOK IS A NONPROFESSIONAL WORK

INFORMING IN EASY WAY ABOUT THE USE OF HERBS,

VITAMINS AND MINERALS FOR MAXIMUM WELL-BEING.

BASED ON SINGLE EXAMPLES,

OR STORIES TOLD BY FAMILY MEMBERS AND FRIENDS

ON HOW EFFECTIVELY SOME PEOPLE

WERE ABLE TO FIGHT OFF SOMETIMES SERIOUS DISEASES.

REMEDIES ARE FROM AROUND THE WORLD,

BUT MOSTLY FROM EASTERN AND WESTERN EUROPE.

TRADITION ON HOW TO USE

HERBS, VITAMINS AND MINERALS ARE CENTURIES OLD.

INFORMATION IN THIS BOOK IS NOT FROM MEDICAL EXPERIENCE,

BUT FROM TRADITIONAL HEALING PRACTICES THAT HAVE BEEN PAST DOWN

FROM GENERATION TO GENERATION.

NOW,

I DO NOT CLAIM TO BE AN EXPERT

ON HOW TO USE HERBS, VITAMINS AND MINERALS FOR HEALING.

I HAVE USED SEVERAL COMBINATIONS

AND SINGLE HERBAL, MINERAL OR VITAMIN

SUPPLEMENTATION.

WHAT I DISCOVERED IS THAT

WHAT WORK FOR ME

MAY NOT WORK FOR SOMEONE ELSE.

THAT IS WHY THERE USUALLY IS

MORE THAN ONE REMEDY FOR ONE PROBLEM

AND YOU NEED TO SEE

WHICH ONE WORKS BEST FOR YOU.

*   *   *

EVERYONE THAT IS WILLING TO USE HERBS, VITAMINS AND MINERALS

IN ORDER TO GET RID OF A HEALTH PROBLEM,

NEED TO TALK TO THEIR DOCTOR.

BECAUSE OF SOME HEALTH CONDITIONS TAKING VITAMIN,

MINERAL OR HERBAL SUPPLEMENTS MAY NOT BE ADVISABLE.

ALSO, OVERDOSE OF SOME VITAMINS AND MINERALS CAN BE TOXIC.

WHEN YOU SUFFER FROM SERIOUS ILLNESS CONSULT YOUR DOCTOR

BEFORE YOU START USING ANY OF NATURAL REMEDIES.

YOU CAN ALSO LOCATE A NATUROPATHIC PHYSICIAN

IN YOUR AREA

(A DOCTOR THAT IS KNOWLEDGEABLE IN NATURAL MEDICINE).

ALL INFORMATION I HAVE ABOUT HERBS, VITAMINS AND MINERALS

I HAVE WRITTEN DOWN IN THIS BOOK,

FOR EVERYONE TO READ AND USE

SO HOPEFULLY SOME SERIOUS ILLNESSES CAN BE AVOIDED . . . .

*   *   *

THERE WILL ALWAYS BE SOMEONE WHO WILL DISAGREE WITH MY WORK

FINDING IT USELESS, PERHAPS.

AND I RESPECT THEIR RIGHT TO DISAGREE.

PERHAPS IT MAY BE USELESS TO MANY,

BECAUSE MANY MAY KNOW ALL THERE IS TO KNOW ABOUT HERBS,
VITAMINS AND MINERALS.

BUT THIS BOOK IS FOR THOSE WHO DON'T KNOW,

AND MAYBE THIS WORK

IS THE ONLY SOURCE ON NATURAL REMEDIES THEY WILL HAVE?

AND IF THIS BOOK WILL HELP AT LEAST ONE PERSON

I FEEL IT WAS WORTH IT FOR ME TO WRITE IT DOWN FOR THIS ONE PERSON . . .

*

ONCE MORE I WOULD LIKE TO MENTION THAT

INFORMATION IN THIS BOOK HAD BEEN WRITTEN

DOWN FROM THE MEMOIRS OF

MY FAMILY AND FRIENDS.

MY MISSION, IS TO PROLONG THE LIFE OF NATURAL

MEDICINE KNOWLEDGE

THAT MY GRANDMOTHERS AND GREAT GRANDMOTHERS

AND THOSE BEFORE THEM

USED IN TIMES WHEN THEY HAD NO ANTIBIOTICS OR PAIN KILLERS . . .

REMEMBER, FOR HERBS TO WORK YOU NEED TO GIVE TIME.

SOME TAKE MONTHS SOME WEEKS.

BE PATIENT.

*　　*　　*

FOR YOUR CONVENIENCE

INFORMATION IS ORGANIZED ALPHABETICALLY.

*

AND ONE LAST THING,

PLEASE DON'T WRITE TO ME FOR ADVICE,

EVERYTHING I KNOW IS IN THIS BOOK.

I DO NOT SELL HERBS OR NATURAL SUPPLEMENTS.

STAY WELL,

LINDA WISE

USE BLANK PAGES FOR NOTES

A

ALCOHOLISM

ANEMIA

ANOREXIA

ARTHRITIS

ANTIOXIDANTS

ANXIETY

ASTHMA

ALCOHOLISM–

ON MANY OCCASIONS I WAS TOLD THAT

IN OLDER TIMES DOCTORS WOULD TREAT ALCOHOLISM WITH VITAMINS.

HOW OFTEN THE TREATMENT SUCCEEDED I DON'T KNOW.

VITAMINS A, D, C AND E WOULD BE ADMINISTERED,

AND ALL OF THE B VITAMINS.

BEFORE YOU START TAKING THE VITAMINS

ASK YOUR DOCTOR ABOUT SAFE DOSES OF THE VITAMINS FOR YOU.

*

ALSO MAGNESIUM SUPPLEMENTS

ARE BENEFICIAL FOR PEOPLE AFFECTED WITH ALCOHOLISM.

—ASK YOUR DOCTOR.

ANEMIA–

EAT PARSLEY GREENS (FRESH)

TAKE DESICCATED LIVER SUPPLEMENTS

EAT THE VEGETABLE—BEETS / ROOT

AND FRESH PAPAYA.

DRINK TEA FROM THE HERB NETTLE.

TAKE B-12 VITAMIN SUPPLEMENT.

REMEMBER,

ALWAYS TALK TO YOUR DOCTOR

WHEN TREATING SERIOUS HEALTH CONDITION.

ANOREXIA–

BREWER'S EAST AND DESICCATED LIVER CONSUMPTION

FOR ABOUT A MONTH.

SUPPLEMENTS OF B VITAMINS

AND GOAT MILK TO DRINK.

THIS WAS THE CURE FOR ANOREXIA

IN OLDER DAYS IN SOME PARTS OF EUROPE.

ANXIETY–

If YOU EXPERIENCE ANXIETY

EAT DIET RICH IN CALCIUM

AND B VITAMINS.

GET ADEQUATE SLEEP.

(READ ALSO ABOUT HYPERACTIVITY).

ARTHRITIS–

To HELP WITH YOUR ARTHRITIS PAINS-

TAKE VITAMIN D SUPPLEMENTS,

OR TRY MAGNESIUM SUPPLEMENT WITH A GLASS OF MILK.

DRINK MANGO JUICE, CHERRY JUICE.

MANGANESE SUPPLEMENT MAY HELP—ASK YOUR DOCTOR,

(MANGANESE SUPPLEMENTS NEED TO BE ADVISED BY DOCTOR).

ALSO TRY

ROSEMARY /HERB—BATH

COOKED WARM CABBAGE LEAF PUT ON HURTING AREA.

ANTIOXIDANTS–

THE BEST ANTIOXIDANTS ARE GRAPE

AND WATERMELON SEEDS.

BITE INTO THE SEEDS AND SWALLOW THEM.

YOU DON'T HAVE TO EAT MANY, ONE OR TWO AT A TIME

WILL DO THE JOB.

DRINK GREEN TEA.

YELLOW ONIONS ARE GREAT SOURCE OF ANTIOXIDANTS.

ASTHMA–

IN OLDER DAYS FOR ASTHMA

PEOPLE WHO SUFFER FROM IT

WOULD BREATH IN THE VAPOR FROM BOILING POTATOES.

ONE WHO SUFFER FROM ASTHMA

SHOULD TAKE SUPPLEMENT MADE FROM CELERY SEED

AND DRINK HYSSOP TEA.

ALSO ASK YOUR DOCTOR ABOUT MAGNESIUM SUPPLEMENTS.

B

BED SORES

BLADDER INFECTIONS

BLEEDING

BONES

(TO HAVE STRONG AND HEALTHY BONES)

BRUISING

(BRUISES, CUTS, SCRAPES)

BED SORES–

YOU COULD GET RID OF BED SORES IN A WEEK.

EAT DIET RICH IN WHEAT GERM AND BREWER'S YEAST,

FRESH FRUITS AND VEGETABLES, MILK AND EGGS,

VITAMIN B-1 AND VITAMIN C.

APPLY OLIVE OIL TOPICALLY.

BLADDER INFECTIONS–

ONE BIG ROOT OF PARSLEY WASH

AND PUT INTO QUART OF WATER

BOIL

LET IT STAND FOR A BOUT 15-20 MINUTES TO

COOL IT DOWN AND DRINK 3 TIMES A DAY

*

TO PREVENT BLADDER INFECTIONS:

USE PARSLEY ROOT FOR YOUR SOUPS AND SALADS

EAT FRESH AND DRIED CRANBERRIES.

DRINK CRANBERRY JUICE.

BLEEDING–

EXCESSIVE BLEEDING

MAY INDICATE

TOO LITTLE VITAMIN K IN THE DIET.

ALSO IF YOU ARE TAKING SUPPLEMENTS OF E VITAMIN

YOU MAY NEED TO STOP FOR A WHILE

IF YOU OBSERVE EXCESSIVE BLEEDING.

ASK YOUR DOCTOR.

BONES–

(TO HAVE STRONG AND HEALTHY BONES)

To HAVE STRONG AND HEALTHY BONES

DRINK LOT'S OF MILK PREFERABLY FROM GOAT.

FOR OLDER FOLKS:

TAKE CALCIUM AND PHOSPHORUS SUPPLEMENTS

CORAL CALCIUM OR BONE MEAL SUPPLEMENTS ARE GOOD.

BONE MEAL INCLUDES PHOSPHORUS.

BRAIN CLARITY–

FOR BRAIN CLARITY AND BETTER MEMORY

TAKE GINGKO BILOBA—HERBAL SUPPLEMENTS.

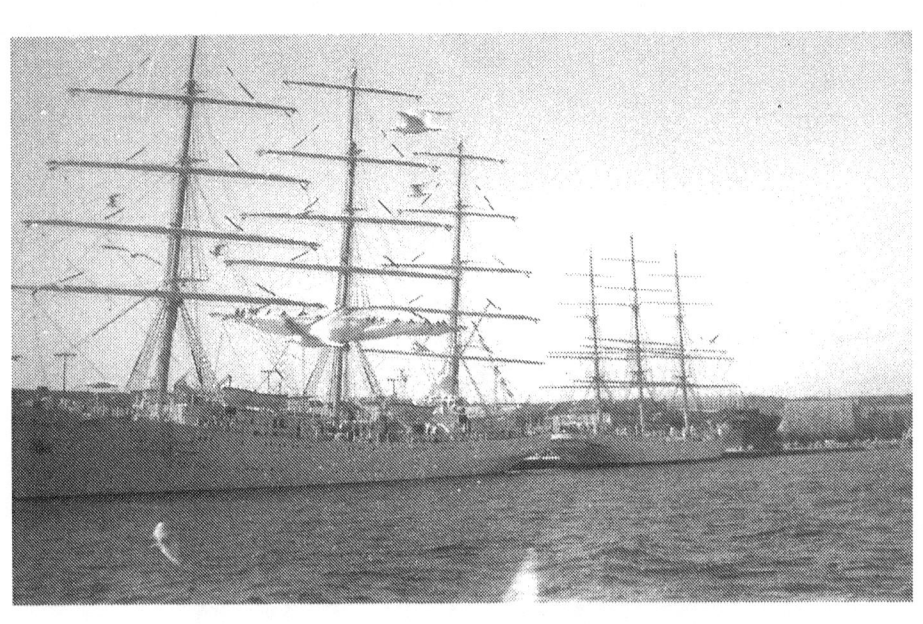

BRUISING–
(BRUISES, CUTS, SCRAPES)

Sign of vitamin c deficiency is bruising.

For scrapes and minor cuts

use the juice of marigold plant.

To minimize scar tissue formation

apply vitamin e topically.

C

CANCER

CANDIDIASIS
(COMMON YEAST INFECTIONS)

CIRCULATION

COMMON COLD AND FLU

CONJUNCTIVITIS

CONSTIPATION

CANCER–

IF YOU HAVE CANCER, FIRST OF ALL

YOU WOULD NEED TO BOOST YOUR IMMUNE SYSTEM.

TO BOOST IMMUNE SYSTEM YOU CAN USE HERBS SUCH AS:

PURPLE CONEFLOWER/ ECHINACEA, LICORICE TEA AND GOLDEN SEAL.

SOME PRACTICAL SUGGESTIONS:

ELIMINATE FRIED FOODS FROM YOUR DIET.

IF YOU MUST EAT FRIED

DO NOT USE DRIPPINGS OR OILS OVER AND OVER AGAIN.

EXERCISE, MAKE YOUR BODY MOVE.

BY DOING THIS, YOU GIVE YOUR BODY CELLS MORE OXYGEN.

(PHYSICAL ACTIVITY I WAS TOLD,

MAY REDUCE YOUR CHANCES TO GET CANCER).

ASK YOUR DOCTOR ABOUT GREEN AND BLUE ALGAE SUPPLEMENTS.

EAT GARLIC, SOME SAY IT SLOWS THE GROWTH OF CANCER,

CAYENNE PEPPER HAS SIMILAR PROPERTIES.

EAT FRESH PEANUTS WITH THE SKINS STILL ON THEM

—DON'T EAT THE SHELLS!

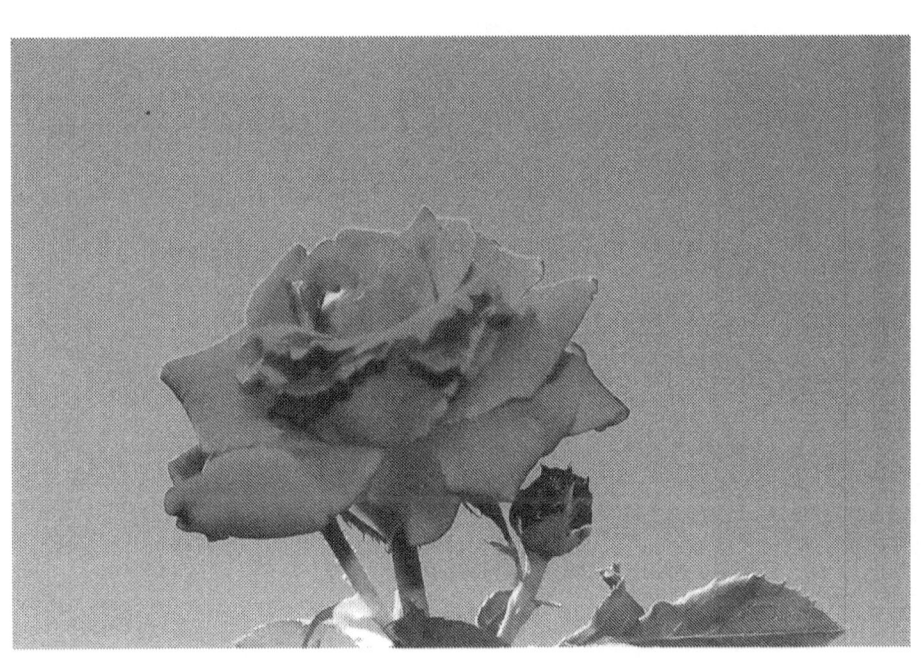

CANCER CONT.

SINCE OLD TIMES, IN FRANCE AND OTHER EUROPEAN COUNTRIES,

SNAILS OF THE NAME ESCARGOTS

HAD BEEN EATEN TO PREVENT BREAST CANCER.

TAKE SUPPLEMENT OF PANAX GINSENG.

*

IF YOU ARE A WOMAN AND NONSMOKER, AND

SUFFER FROM LUNG CANCER,

TRY TO EAT A SNAIL OF THE NAME ULEX EUROPEUS.

*

INTRODUCE GRAIN AMARANTH TO YOUR DIET TO AVOID COLON CANCER.

CANDIDIASIS–

CANDIDIASIS IS ANOTHER NAME FOR COMMON YEAST INFECTION.

IF YOU SUFFER FROM IT, CUT DOWN ON SUGAR

AND WHEAT PRODUCTS.

AVOID WHOLE GRAIN BREADS.

EAT YOGURT WITH ACTIVE L. ACIDOPHILUS CULTURES

CIRCULATION–

For BETTER CIRCULATION TAKE

HAWTHORN BERRIES /HERBAL SUPPLEMENTS

AND OMEGA 3 SUPPLEMENTS.

TO PREVENT STROKE, EAT PLENTY OF:

NUTS, LIVER, GREEN LEAFY VEGETABLES,

VITAMIN E FOODS.

*

EXERCISE PREFERABLY OUTDOORS, TAKE LONG WALKS

(BY MOVING YOUR BODY

YOU ARE HELPING YOUR HEART

TO PUSH YOUR BLOOD AROUND YOUR BODY).

IN OLDER DAYS PEOPLE HAD TO MOVE AROUND MORE THAN TODAY,

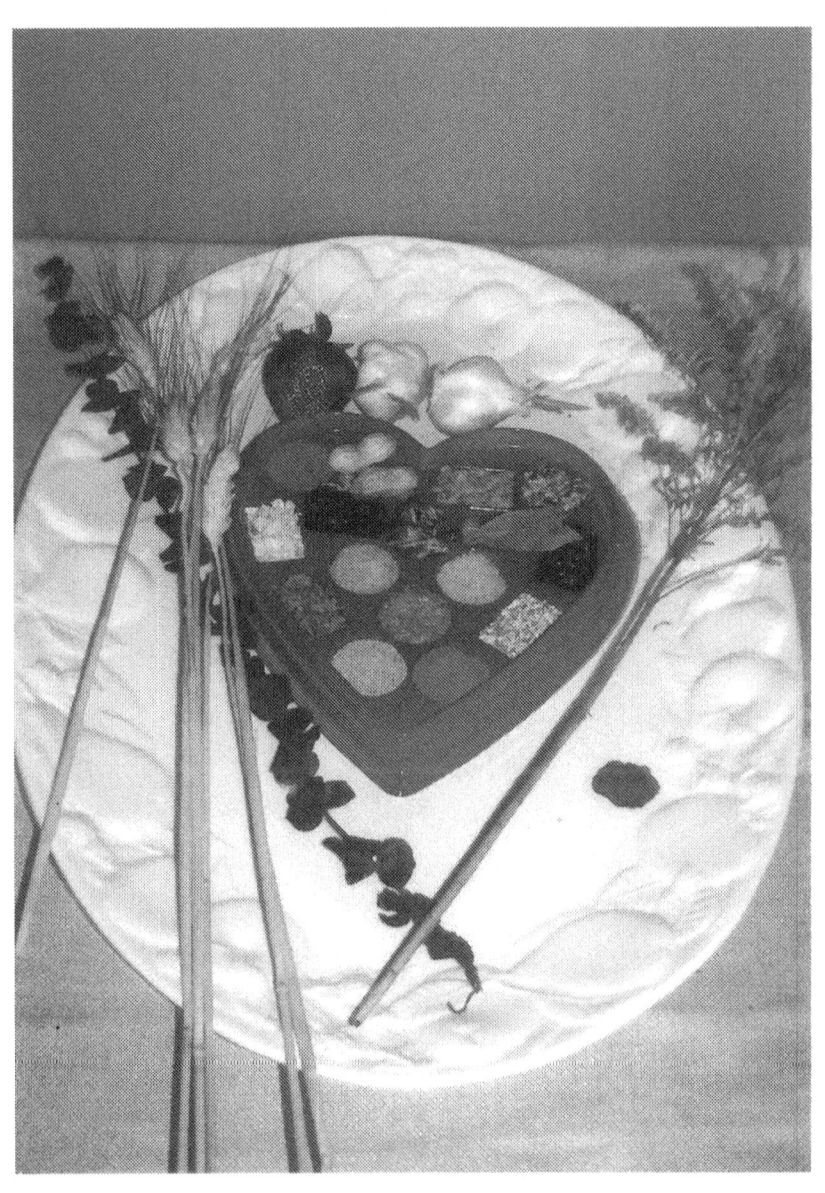

CIRCULATION CONT.

THEY HAD TO DO THINGS FOR THEMSELVES,

THEY GATHERED FOOD, CAME HOME

AND COOKED THE FOOD, AND THEY HAD NO TELEVISION . . .

THEY USUALLY MOVED CONSTANTLY . . .

LET IT BE A LESSON FOR US.

IT WAS A GOOD THING FOR THE HEART.

COMMON COLD AND FLU–

REMEMBER IS EASIER TO PREVENT, THEN TREAT.

*

DRINK LICORICE TEA AND GOLDEN SEAL TEA.

PURPLE CONEFLOWER IS KNOWN TO BOOST IMMUNE SYSTEM.

TAKE VITAMINS WITH ZINC TO PREVENT COLDS AND FLU

EAT PLENTY OF FRUITS AND VEGETABLES FOR VITAMIN C.

HUMIDIFIER HELPS WITH THE DRYNESS IN YOUR NOSE AND THROAT.

WASH YOUR HANDS OFTEN.

IS GOOD TO OPEN WINDOW FOR A WHILE

TO REFRESH THE AIR IN YOUR ROOM.

*

VITAMIN A IS IMPORTANT FOR THE PREVENTION OF INFECTIONS.

EAT PLENTY OF APRICOTS, CARROTS AND EGG YOLK.

COMMON COLD AND FLU CONT.

*

MAKE YOUR OWN ONION COUGH SYRUP:

SLICE MEDIUM SIZE YELLOW ONION,

PUT IN A SMALL JAR.

USE 5 OR 6 TABLE SPOONS OF SUGAR

TO COVER THE ONION.

CLOSE THE JAR AND PUT IT IN A SUNNY SPOT.

THE HEAT FROM THE SUN WILL JUICE THE ONION

AND TOGETHER WITH THE SUGAR

IT WILL MAKE RATHER TASTY COUGH SYRUP

AND EFFECTIVE TOO!

*

CONSTIPATION–

Eat prunes or drink prune juice.

Eat fresh pineapple.

Severe constipation

may be the result of B vitamins deficiency

-talk to your doctor.

D

DEPRESSION

DIARRHEA

DIABETES

DEPRESSION–

PEOPLE WHO SUFFER FROM DEPRESSION MAY LACK B VITAMINS.

THEY MAY ALSO HAVE MAGNESIUM DEFICIENCY.

EAT PLENTY OF FRESH FRUITS AND VEGETABLES.

IF YOU SUFFER FROM DEPRESSION,

TAKE VACATION IF POSSIBLE

OR DO SOMETHING EXCLUSIVELY FOR YOURSELF—

LIKE RELAXING MASSAGE . . .

OR GO TO A MOVIE THEATER—
SEE A GOOD COMEDY.

OUR SURROUNDINGS ARE VERY IMPORTANT TO OUR MOOD

AND RELAXATION.

TAKE ADEQUATE SLEEP.

WEAR COLORFUL CLOTHES!

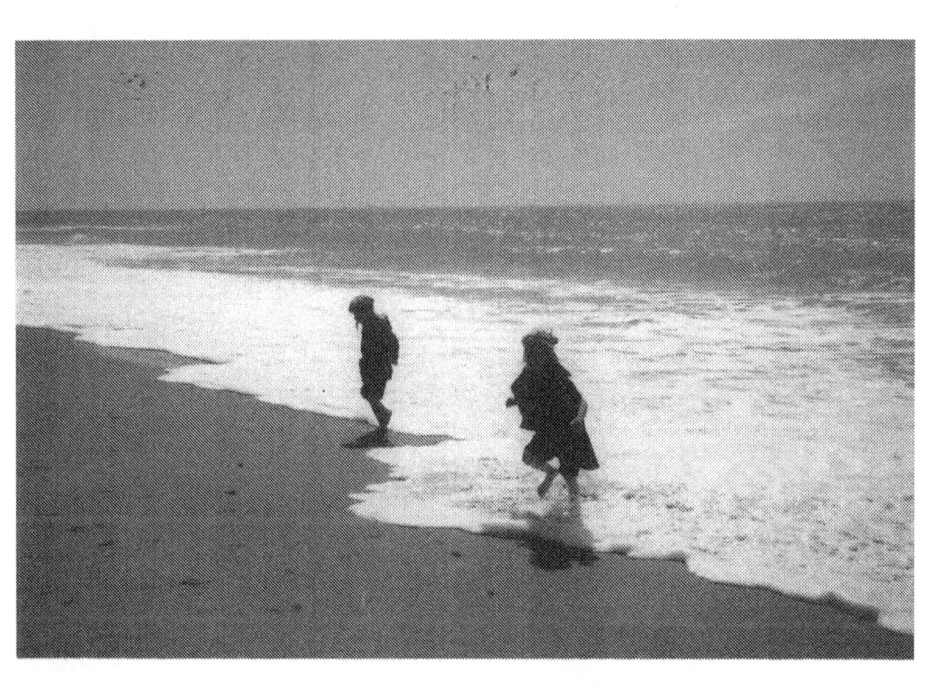

DIARRHEA–

To stop diarrhea

eat:

Bananas and blueberries

restrict fruit juice.

Eat vegetable and meaty soups,

and plain white bread toast.

DIABETES–

PEOPLE WHO SUFFER FROM DIABETES

SHOULD BE TAKING FISH LIVER OIL SUPPLEMENT

TO PREVENT NIGHT BLINDNESS.

ASK YOUR DOCTOR ABOUT VITAMIN E SUPPLEMENTATION.

E

EARACHE

EAR INFECTIONS

EDEMA (SWELLING)

EYES

EARACHE–

FOR EARACHE USE

EUCALYPTUS OIL EAR DROP OR

GARLIC MULLEIN OLIVE OIL EAR DROP

EAR INFECTIONS–

To PREVENT EAR INFECTION IN CHILDREN,

CHILDREN'S VITAMIN WITH ZINC SHOULD BE GIVEN

ESPECIALLY IN THE WINTER MONTHS.

CUT DOWN ON DIARY PRODUCTS AND AVOID

CORN INTAKE TO MINIMIZE THE CHANCES OF GETTING EAR INFECTION.

. . . ALSO CUT DOWN ON SUGAR.

EDEMA–
(SWELLING)

DEFICIENCY IN MAGNESIUM CAN CAUSE EDEMA.

ALSO THE CAUSE OF SWELLING

CAN BE MALFUNCTION OF THE KIDNEYS,

—READ ABOUT KIDNEYS.

EYES–

FOR "PINK EYE" (CONJUNCTIVITIS) TRY SLICE OF FRESH TOMATO.

FRESH SLICE PUT ON THE EYE AND HOLD FOR FEW SECONDS,

REPEAT IF NECESSARY

(THE JUICE FROM THE TOMATO DOES NOT HURT YOUR EYE

AND IS NEEDED TO HELP WITH THE PROBLEM).

I HAVE BEEN USING THE TOMATO CURE

ALSO FOR OCCASIONAL EYE DRYNESS

—WITH SUCCESS.

BURNING SENSATION IN YOUR EYE?

TRY TOMATO SLICE.

THE SUN VITAMIN—VITAMIN D

MAY PREVENT NEARSIGHTEDNESS IN CHILDREN.

DRYNESS AND BURNING OF THE EYES

MAY BE THE RESULT OF B VITAMINS DEFICIENCY

-CHECK WITH YOUR DOCTOR.

EYES CONT.

FOR BURNING SENSATIONS IN YOUR EYES CHECK IF THE

CHLORINE IN YOUR WATER IS NOT THE TROUBLE MAKER.

-TURN TO BOTTLED WATER IF

THAT'S THE CASE.

DRYNESS AND BURNING OF YOUR EYES-

WATCH THE FRESH FRUITS YOU EAT,

SOME MAY NEED TO BE PEELED BEFORE YOU CONSUME THEM.

VITAMIN A DEFICIENCY RESULTS IN . . . . NIGHT BLINDNESS.

IF IT IS UNCOMFORTABLE FOR YOU TO GO OUTSIDE

IN BRIGHT SUNSHINE WITHOUT SUNGLASSES,

THEN MOST LIKELY YOU ARE SHORT ON VITAMIN A.

*

EAT FRESH SUNFLOWER SEEDS FOR GOOD VISION.

FISH LIVER OIL SUPPLEMENT FOR YOUNG AND OLD

IS A NATURAL FOOD FOR VITAMIN A

TAKEN FROM THE LIVERS OF COD, HALIBUT, ETC.

YOU CAN ALSO EAT FOR VITAMIN A

FOODS SUCH AS:

APRICOTS, CARROTS, BEEF LIVER, EGG YOLK, SWEET POTATOES.

F

FATIGUE

FEET

FUNGUS
(NAIL FUNGUS)

FATIGUE–

IF YOU SUFFER FROM FATIGUE,

DRINK LICORICE TEA.

TAKE GINSENG SUPPLEMENTS AND

USE CAYENNE PEPPER TO SPICE UP YOUR SALADS AND SOUPS.

SUPPLEMENT OF B VITAMINS MAY BE NEEDED.

EAT PLENTY OF FRESH FRUITS AND VEGETABLES

YOU MAY NEED MAGNESIUM SUPPLEMENTATION

-ASK YOUR DOCTOR

FEET–

To PREVENT BURNING FEET SENSATION

EAT B VITAMINS IN YOUR FOOD.

FOODS IN WHICH VITAMIN B IS PLENTIFUL ARE:

LEGUMES, ORGAN MEATS (HEART, LIVER, KIDNEYS),

SOYBEANS, EGG YOLK

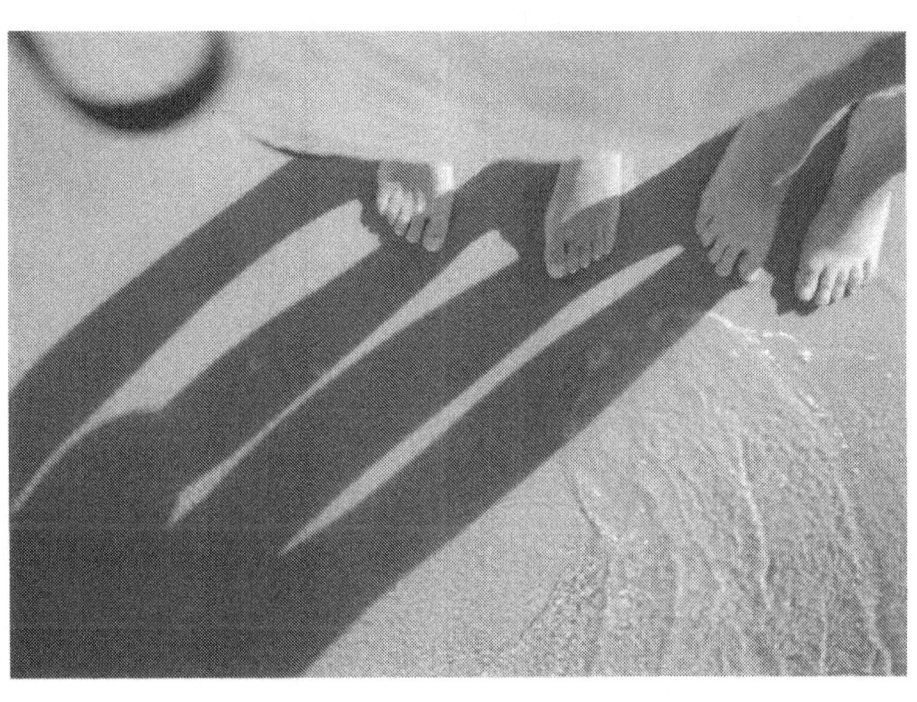

FUNGUS–
(NAIL FUNGUS)

IF YOU HAVE FUNGUS ON YOUR TOE NAILS

SOAK YOUR FEET IN SALTY WATER, THE MORE SALT THE BETTER.

REPEAT DAILY,

SOAK FOR 15 MINUTES OR SO.

YOU CAN ALSO USE HYDROGEN PEROXIDE TO WASH YOUR NAILS WITH.

REPEAT EVERY DAY UNTIL YOUR NAILS ARE WHITE.

IF YOUR NAILS ARE YELLOW COLOR

USE HYDROGEN PEROXIDE TO SOAK YOUR NAILS IN.

G

GUMS

GUMS–

FOR GUMS TO STOP BLEEDING

EAT SUNFLOWER SEEDS (FRESH)

DO NOT CHEW ON ONE SIDE OF YOUR MOUTH ONLY

IT IS IMPORTANT

TO USE BOTH SIDES OF YOUR MOUTH EVENLY WHEN CHEWING.

SPONGY GUMS TO THE TOUCH AND BLEEDING?

CONSUME MORE VITAMIN C.

TENDER GUMS?

YOU MAY NEED B VITAMINS SUPPLEMENTATION

—ASK YOUR DOCTOR

H

HAIR–

LOSS OF HAIR?

MAYBE MAGNESIUM AND CALCIUM DEFICIENCY.

HAIR THAT IS BRITTLE, DRY AND OFTEN FULL OF DANDRUFF

—THESE ARE SIGNS OF VITAMIN A DEFICIENCY.

PREMATURE GREY HAIR,

PERHAPS IRON AND COPPER DEFICIENCY?

ASK YOUR DOCTOR ABOUT SAFE DOSES OF THIS SUPPLEMENTS FOR YOU.

AND REMEMBER SUPPLEMENTATION IN NATURAL FORM IS THE BEST.

*

-TALK TO YOUR DOCTOR ABOUT SUPPLEMENTATION,

SOME SUPPLEMENTS NEED TO BE TAKEN IN VERY SMALL AMOUNTS.

REMEMBER OVERDOSE OF SOME SUPPLEMENTS CAN BE TOXIC!

HEADACHES–

To GET RID OF HEADACHES USE THE HERB:

STONE ROOT.

EAT PLAIN WHITE BREAD TOAST AND REDUCE INTAKE OF SALT.

REMEMBER, CONTINUED USE OF SOME MEDICATIONS

CAN ACTUALLY PRODUCE HEADACHE.

DON'T BE HABITUAL USER OF MEDICATIONS.

YOU MAY THINK

THAT YOU ARE TAKING THIS PARTICULAR MEDICINE

TO HELP YOURSELF WITH HEADACHE,

BUT IN REALITY THE MEDICINE MAY CAUSE THE HEADACHE.

SOME FOLKS BECAME ADDICTED TO SOME MEDICINES

THEY HAVE NOT EVEN REALIZED THEY DO NOT NEED THEM REALLY . . .

TALK TO YOUR DOCTOR.

IF YOU HAVE REPEATED HEADACHES

CHECK IF YOU ARE PERHAPS ALLERGIC TO SOME FOODS.

SOME PEOPLE WHO EXPERIENCE REPEATED HEADACHES

ARE ALLERGIC TO DUST.

HEARING–

Sinuses and ears are affected

when there is an excess of salt in the body.

I had been told stories of deaf people who

by giving up salt had regain hearing.

Reduce also intake of

other fluid retention foods

such as sodium and sugar.

HEART–

Hawthorn berries / herb.

HAWTHORN BERRIES IS AN HERB

MY WHOLE FAMILY AND FRIENDS TAKE IT DAILY.

IF YOU HAVE A HISTORY OF HEART PROBLEMS

THIS HERB IS HIGHLY EFFECTIVE.

TAKE ALSO VITAMIN E, OMEGA 3 SUPPLEMENTS,

OR EAT FOODS RICH IN OMEGA 3

SUCH AS: SARDINES, SALMON, COD, ETC.,

EAT OATS/OATMEAL.

*

TAKE WALKS FOR YOUR HEART.

ALWAYS TALK TO YOUR DOCTOR ABOUT ANY SUPPLEMENTS

YOU ARE TAKING, IF YOU HAVE HEART PROBLEM.

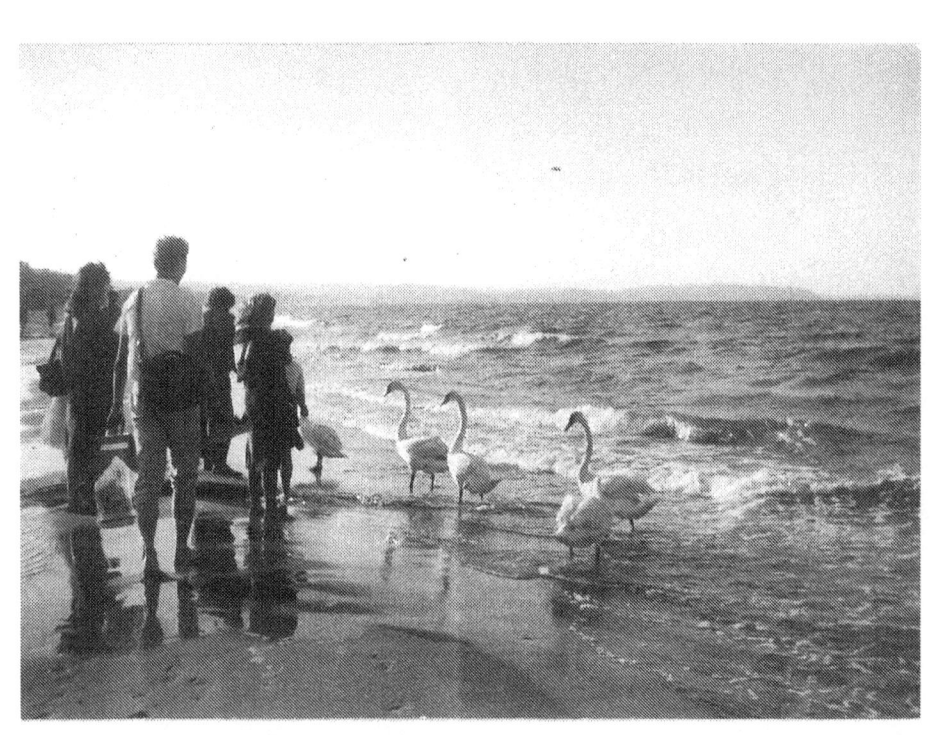

HYPERACTIVITY–

For hyperactivity use

herbal teas:

chamomile, valerian or licorice tea.

hyperactivity maybe result of magnesium

and b vitamins deficiency—ask your doctor.

I

IMMUNE SYSTEM
(TO BOOST IMMUNE SYSTEM)

IMMUNE SYSTEM–

(TO BOOST IMMUNE SYSTEM)

IF YOU HAVE STRONG IMMUNE SYSTEM

YOU CAN FIGHT OFF MANY SERIOUS ILLNESSES ON YOUR OWN.

*

DO YOU SUFFER FROM A SERIOUS ILLNESS?

IF YOU DO

YOUR GOAL SHOULD BE

TO GET YOUR IMMUNE SYSTEM IN GOOD SHAPE.

I WILL WRITE DOWN EVERYTHING I HAVE HEARD

ABOUT BOOSTING AN IMMUNE SYSTEM.

*

TAKE SUPPLEMENTS OR DRINK TEA

FROM HERB PURPLE CONE FLOWER.

DRINK LICORICE TEA AND GREEN TEA.

EAT PINEAPPLE AND GRAPES WITH THE SEEDS IN THEM,

ONE OR TWO SEEDS WILL DO,

BUT BITE THE SEEDS AND SWALLOW.

USE YELLOW ONIONS IN YOUR COOKING AND EAT GARLIC.

EAT VITAMIN C IN YOUR FOODS DAILY.

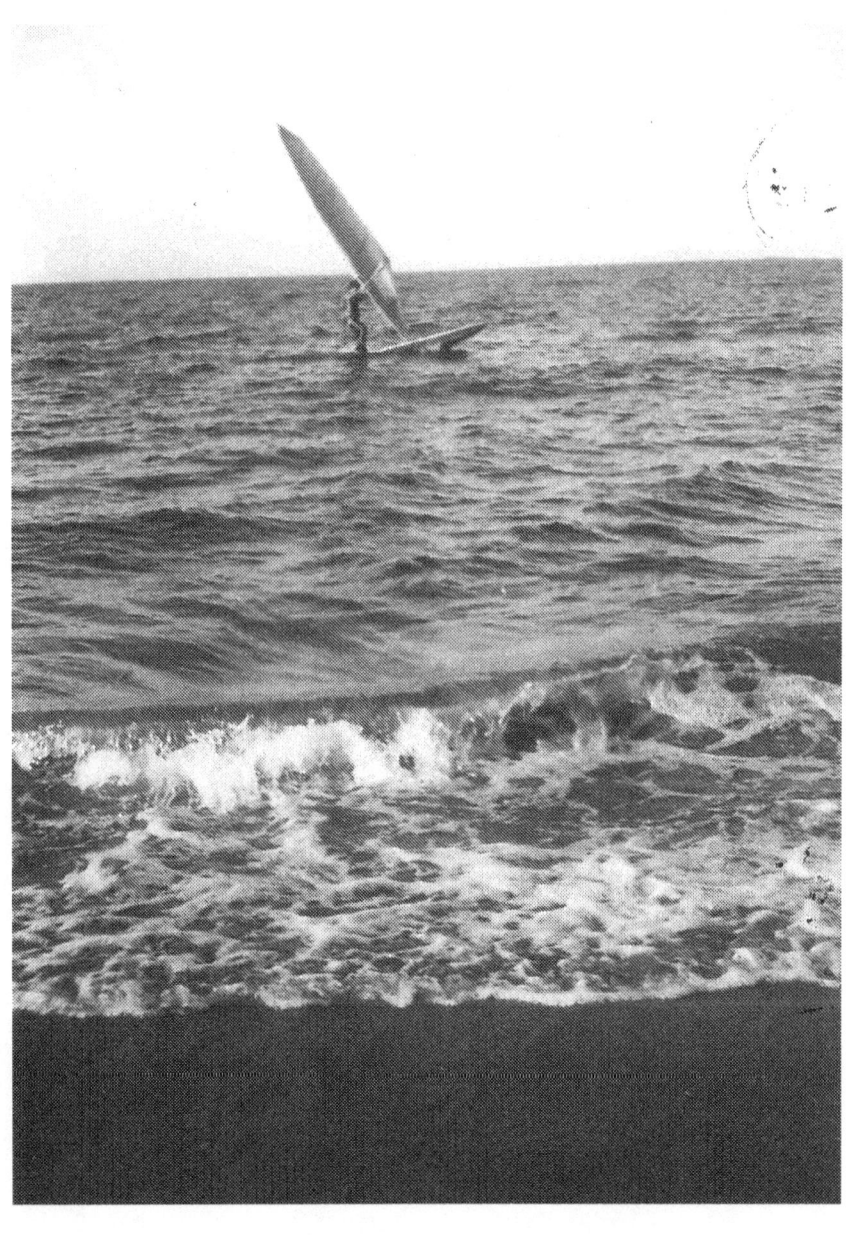

INFERTILITY AND MISCARRIAGES–

DEFICIENCY IN VITAMIN E

AND STRESS MAYBE THE REASON OF INFERTILITY.

TO AVOID MISCARRIAGES

TAKE VITAMIN C + BIOFLAVONOIDS.

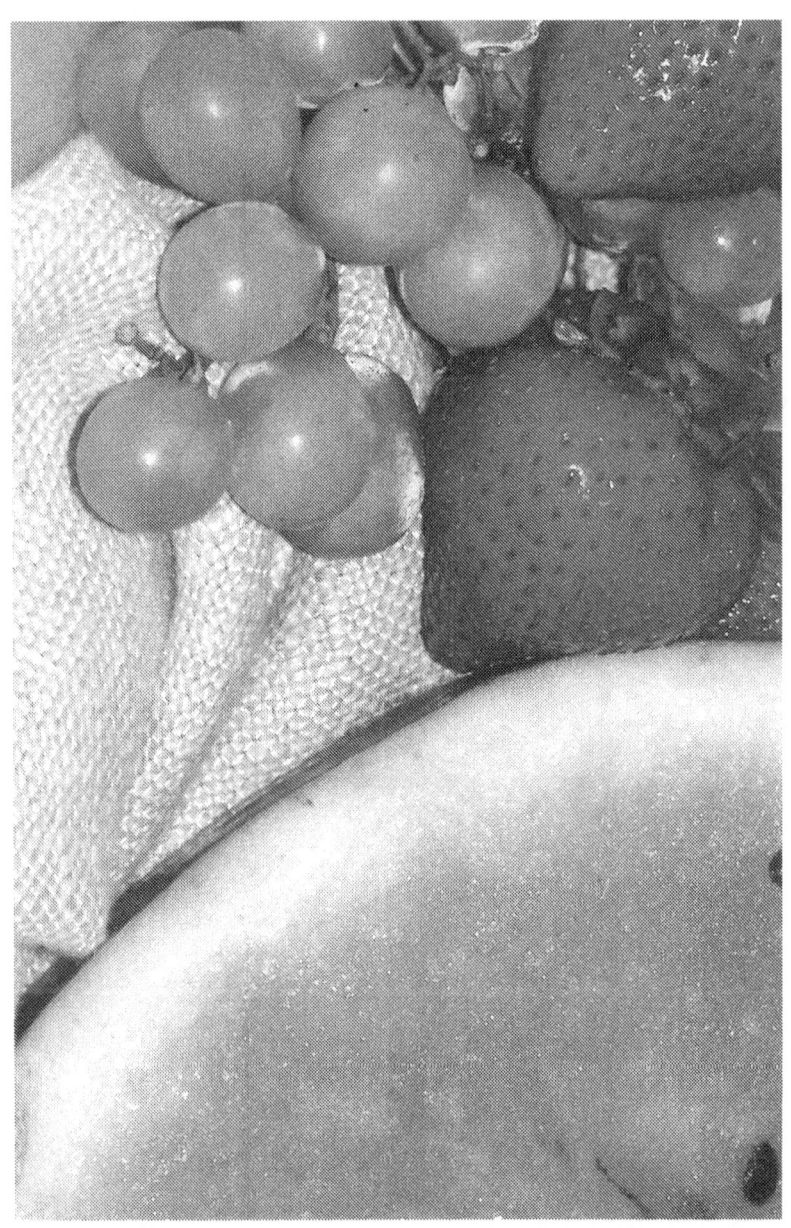

INTESTINAL DISORDERS–

For mild intestinal disorders

eat fresh garlic

and fresh pineapple.

J

JOINTS PAIN

JAUNDICE

JOINTS PAIN–

WHEN JOINTS HURT,

ASK YOUR DOCTOR IF YOU COULD GET MANGANESE SUPPLEMENT.

DRINK CHERRY AND MANGO JUICE.

TAKE MAGNESIUM SUPPLEMENTS WITH A GLASS OF MILK.

ALSO TAKE SUPPLEMENT OF OMEGA 3

(FOR OMEGA 3—EAT SARDINES,

SALMON AND USE FLAX SEED OIL).

JAUNDICE–

To GET RID OF JAUNDICE DRINK JUICE

FROM PLANT CHELIDONIUM MAJUS

(COMMON NAME SWALLOW WART).

*

ALWAYS CONSULT YOUR DOCTOR.

K

KIDNEYS

KIDNEYS–

KIDNEY DAMAGE MAYBE RESULT OF MAGNESIUM DEFICIENCY.

FOR THE HEALTH OF YOUR KIDNEYS DRINK CRANBERRY JUICE

AND EAT FRESH AND DRY CRANBERRIES.

AS NATURAL DIURETIC YOU CAN USE

CELERY SEED AND CELERY THE VEGETABLE.

ALSO FRESH DILL.

DRINK GREEN TEA AND CORNSILK TEA.

TO GET RID OF KIDNEY STONES

USE CAYENNE PEPPER IN YOUR COOKING.

IF YOUR EYES ARE PUFFY

AND YOU HAVE DARK CIRCLES AROUND YOUR EYES

TRY GOLDEN SEAL /HERBAL TEA.

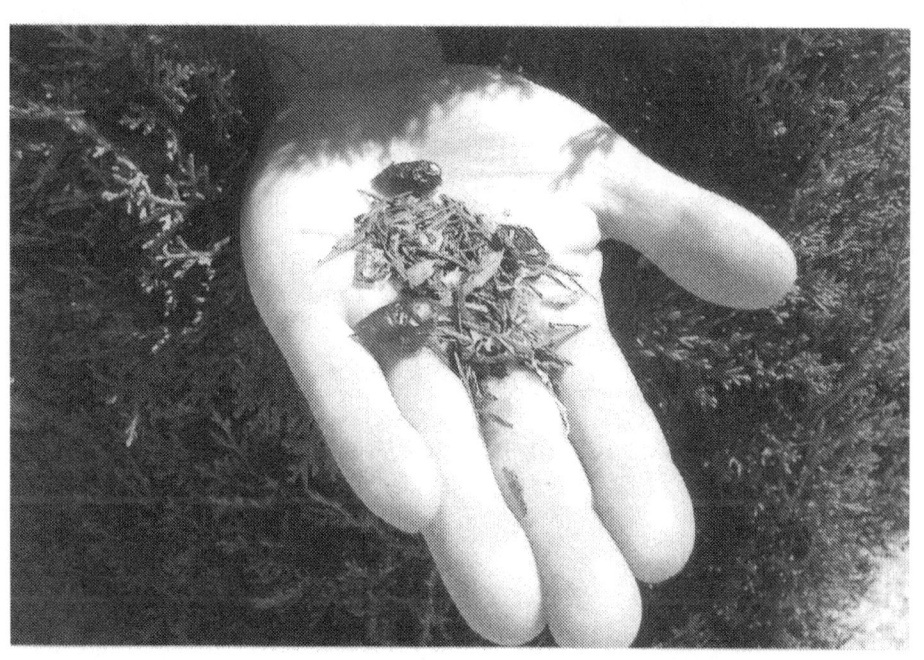

KIDNEYS CONT.

NOW REMEMBER YOU SHOULD NOT DRINK THIS TEA FOR

LONGER THAN A WEEK.

THIS ARE CENTURY OLD REMEDIES

AND PEOPLE BEEN USING THEM FOR VERY LONG TIME . . . .

NEVER THE LESS ALWAYS CONSULT YOUR DOCTOR

WHEN TRYING TO TREAT SERIOUS HEALTH CONDITION.

L

LIPS

LIVER DISEASE

LONGEVITY

LUNGS

LIPS–

For beautiful lips,

women would massage their lips

with the skins from citrus fruit.

LIVER DISEASE–

IF YOU SUFFER FROM LIVER DISEASE

DRINK LICORICE TEA

(I DO NOT KNOW EXACTLY

WHAT IT DOES, BUT IS VERY GOOD TO YOUR LIVER).

TAKE SUPPLEMENTS OF THE HERB MILK TISTLE.

USE YELLOW ONIONS IN YOUR COOKING.

THERAPIES FOR LIVER PROBLEMS IN OLDER TIMES

INCLUDED LARGE PORTIONS OF FRESH LIVER FROM SHEEP

AND COW.

AN HERB CALLED CELANDINE OR MORE COMMONLY SWALLOW WART

HELPS TO CLEAN YOUR LIVER.

LONGEVITY–

CONSUME CALVES LIVER AND OTHER FOODS

THAT CAN GIVE VITAMIN A TO YOU.

(IN NATURAL FORM ONLY—NO SYNTHETIC SUPPLEMENTS)

FOR STRENGTH TAKE—WHEAT GERM.

EAT LOTS OF SOUPS.

USE OLIVE OIL.

REDUCE CONSUMPTION OF POTATOES, INCLUDE MORE RICE.

AVOID STRESS.

INCREASE THE SOURCE OF VITAMIN C IN YOUR DIET.

DON'T USE ANTIBIOTICS INDISCRIMINATELY.

EXERCISE AND SPENT TIME OUTDOORS.

GET ADEQUATE REST.

AVOID POLLUTANTS AND PESTICIDES.

LUNGS–

IF THERE IS TROUBLE WITH YOUR LUNGS,

YOU MAY WANT TO TAKE SUPPLEMENTS MADE

FROM GREEN AND BLUE ALGAE.

ASK YOUR DOCTOR.

M

MENSTRUAL PROBLEMS

MOSQUITO BITES

MOUTH

MULTIPLE SCLEROSIS

MUSCULAR DYSTROPHY

MENOPAUSE–

To FIGHT SEVERE SYMPTOMS OF MENOPAUSE

EAT SOYBEANS AND YAMS.

USE FLAX SEED OIL FOR YOUR SOUPS AND SALADS.

FOR MOOD SWINGS ASSOCIATED WITH MENOPAUSE TAKE

BLACK COHOSH/ HERB—SUPPLEMENTS.

LOOK FOR PHYTOESTROGENS

(SUPPLEMENTS MADE FROM PLANTS)

IN YOUR LOCAL HEALTH FOOD STORE,

THEY PROVED TO BE HIGHLY EFFECTIVE.

ALWAYS DISCUSS YOUR SYMPTOMS WITH YOUR DOCTOR.

MENSTRUAL PROBLEMS–

For IRREGULARITY OF YOUR MENSTRUAL CYCLES

AND PAIN,

TAKE THE HERB JAMAICAN DOGWOOD

AND BLACK COHOSH.

MOSQUITO BITES–

To AVOID MOSQUITO BITES STOP EATING SWEET FOODS

ABOUT ONE MONTH BEFORE MOSQUITO SEASON STARTS.

IF MOSQUITO BITES ARE EXCESSIVE YOU MAY BE LACKING B VITAMINS.

*

DON'T USE SWEET SMELLING DEODORANTS

ON YOUR SKIN

AND WEAR PROTECTIVE CLOTHING.

MOUTH–

CRACKS AT THE CORNERS OF THE MOUTH ?

TRY TO EAT FOODS SUCH AS:

LEGUMES, WHEAT GERM, ORGAN MEATS (KIDNEYS, HEART, LIVER),

EGG YOLK OR SOYBEANS.

THESE ARE THE FOODS IN WHICH VITAMIN B IS MOST PLENTIFUL.

MULTIPLE SCLEROSIS–

For MULTIPLE SCLEROSIS

TAKE GINGKO BILOBA AND DRINK

GOLDEN SEAL AND

LICORICE TEA.

YOU CAN FIND THIS SUPPLEMENTS IN YOUR HEALTH FOOD STORE.

ALWAYS TALK TO YOUR DOCTOR

ABOUT SUPPLEMENTS YOU ARE PLANNING TO TAKE.

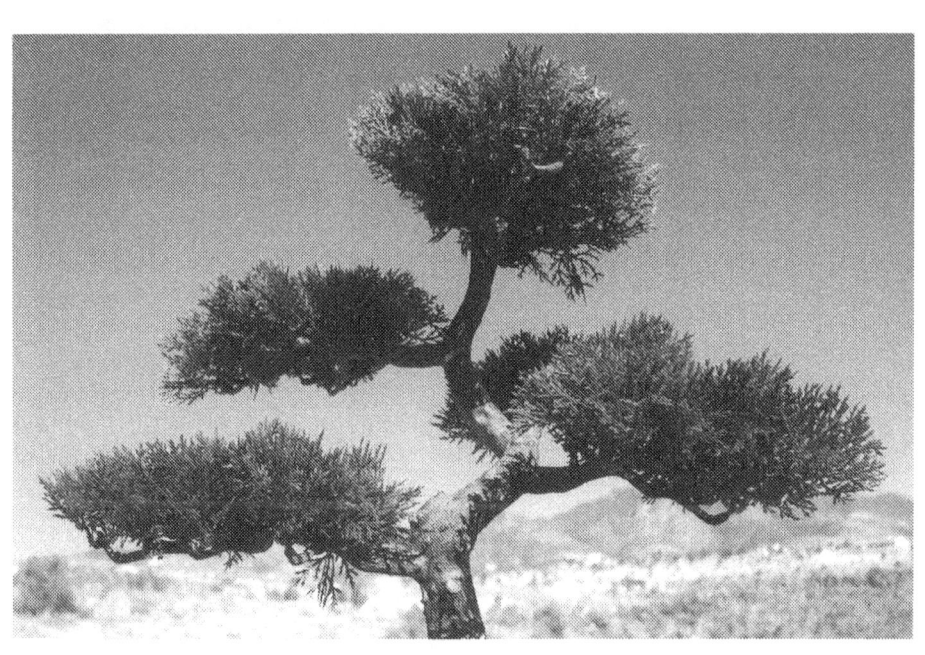

MUSCULAR DYSTROPHY–

I HAVE BEEN TOLD ABOUT SUCCESSFUL TREATMENTS

OF MUSCULAR DYSTROPHY

THAT INVOLVED SUPPLEMENTS OF VITAMIN E AND WHEAT GERM.

-TALK TO YOUR DOCTOR.

N

NAILS

NAILS–

ARE YOUR NAILS BRITTLE AND THIN ?

SOAK THEM IN OLIVE OIL FOR 15-20 MINUTES

THEN WASH OFF THE EXCESS OF OIL WITH WARM WATER.

IF YOUR NAILS ARE YELLOW, SOAK THEM IN HYDROGEN PEROXIDE

REPEAT DAILY UNTIL WHITE.

*

IF YOU OBSERVE WHITE SPOTS ON YOUR NAILS,

THAT MAY BE INDICATION OF B VITAMIN DEFICIENCY.

IN CHILDREN WHITE SPOTS

ALSO INDICATE CALCIUM DEFICIENCY.

O

OSTEOPOROSIS

OVERWEIGHT

OSTEOPOROSIS–

IF YOU HAVE OSTEOPOROSIS

EAT CANNED SALMON AND SARDINES WITH BONES.

TAKE BONE MEAL (CALCIUM AND PHOSPHORUS) SUPPLEMENTS.

EAT FRESH BANANAS.

OVERWEIGHT–
(NOT FROM ILLNESS)

CAREFUL SELECTION OF FOODS

IS REALLY THE SOURCE OF HEALTHY BODY WEIGHT.

EAT FRESH FRUITS AND VEGETABLES.

AVOID FRIED FOODS! AND CARBONATED DRINKS!

LIMIT SODIUM AND SUGAR INTAKE.

CONSUME FRESH GARLIC DAILY.

EAT PLENTY OF FRESH PINEAPPLE.

EXERCISE.

TAKE LONG WALKS.

REMEMBER,

POSITIVE ATTITUDE AND DETERMINATION IS HALF OF YOUR SUCCESS!

P

PARALYSIS

PARASITES

POTENT HEALING
(IN MEN)

PROSTATE GLAND TROUBLES

PULSE

PARALYSIS–

I HAVE HEARD SO MANY WONDERFUL EXAMPLES OF HEALING

WITH HERBS, VITAMINS AND MINERALS . . .

*

BUT REMEMBER,

NOT ALWAYS YOU CAN COUNT ON NATURAL REMEDY TO GET RID OF
YOUR PROBLEM

ESPECIALLY WHEN YOUR CONDITION IS SEVERE, BUT IS WORTH TRYING.

*

ONE OF MY FAVORITES IS ABOUT SOMEONE WHO

HAD BEEN CURED OF LOWER BODY PARALYSIS.

THE PATIENT WAS GIVEN VITAMIN B1 AND VITAMIN C

IN ADDITION TO A DIET

THAT STRESSED WHEAT GERM, FRESH VEGETABLES, PAPAYA, EGGS

AND MILK.

PARASITES–

TO GET RID OF PARASITES, BACTERIA AND VIRUSES

DRINK GOLDEN SEAL AND LICORICE ROOT TEA.

TO GET RID OF PARASITES EXCLUSIVELY :

DRINK THE WATER FROM THE KOSHER DILLS

YOU BUY AT YOUR SUPERMARKET.

DRINK THE JUICE FROM SAUERKRAUT

OR EAT THE VEGETABLE BEET.

YOU CAN ALSO EAT HEARRING FILLETS IN VINEGAR.

*

NOW,

ONE MORE OF THE OLD EASTERN EUROPEAN REMEDY SAYS :

DRINK CUP OF WARM MILK

WITH MEDIUM SIZE GARLIC CLOVE

AND ONE TEA SPOON OF HONEY.

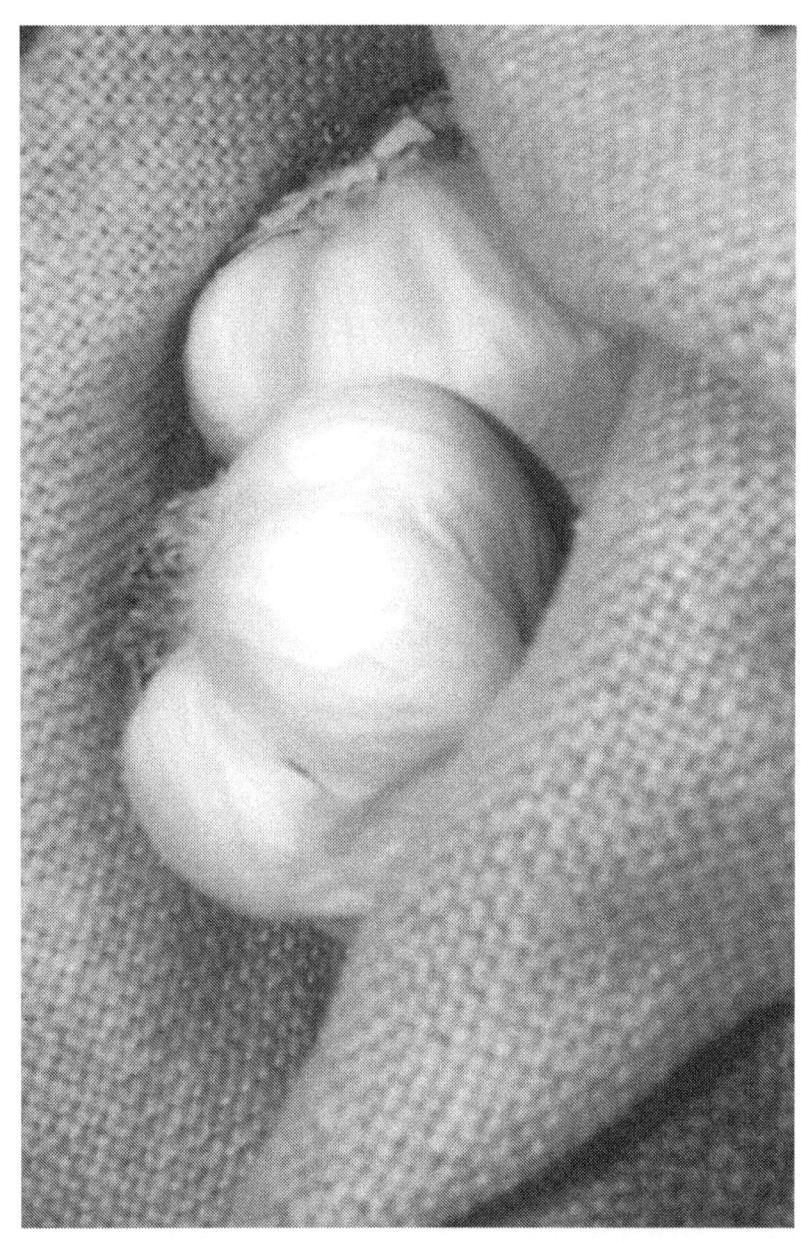

POTENT HEALING–

(IN MEN)

THE MUSHROOM OF THE NAME MAITAKE

(I BELIEVE NATIVE OF JAPAN)

HAD BEEN EATEN TO HEAL POTENCY IN MEN.

IN OLD TIMES IN ROMANIA AND SURROUNDING REGIONS

PUMPKIN SEEDS HAD BEEN EATEN FOR THE SAME REASON.

PROSTATE GLAND TROUBLES–

Eating of pumpkin seeds

has a beneficial effect

on the health of the prostate gland.

To prevent prostate trouble

eat unprocessed seeds like peanuts.

Eat whole grains and take fish liver oil supplements.

Eat garlic, mustard seeds, spinach and broccoli.

Also cooked tomato

like in spaghetti sauce, pizza or tomato soup.

And eat cabbage soup.

PULSE–

TO HAVE GOOD PULSE TAKE SUPPLEMENTS MADE FROM:

HAWTHORN BERRIES / HERB.

*

SOME FOODS MAY AFFECT YOUR PULSE.

WATCH WHAT YOU EAT.

WHOLE WHEAT AND FRIED FOODS

ARE THE USUALLY TROUBLE MAKERS.

R

REPRODUCTIVE DISORDERS
(IN WOMEN)

RHEUMATIC FEVER

RHEUMATISM

REPRODUCTIVE DISORDERS–

(IN WOMEN)

VITAMIN E DEFICIENCY AND STRESS IN SOME PEOPLES

MAY BE THE REASON OF:

INFERTILITY, MISCARRIAGES AND

MENSTRUAL DISORDERS.

*

EAT LOTS OF VITAMIN C

AND BIOFLAVONOIDS

TO AVOID REPEATED MISCARRIAGES.

RHEUMATIC FEVER–

RHEUMATIC FEVER MAYBE CONDITIONED BY EGG CONSUMPTION.

(USE ORGANIC EGGS).

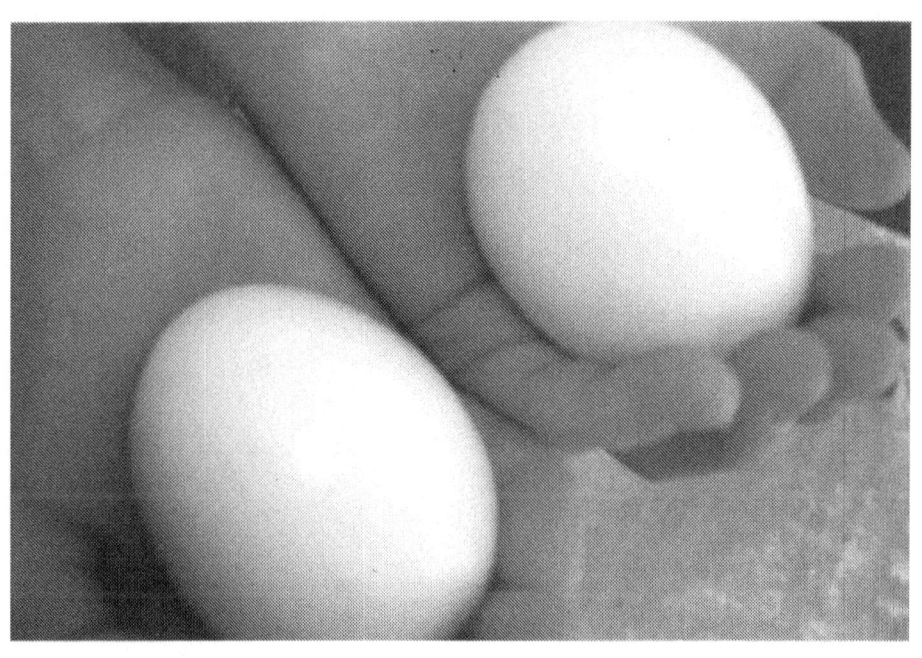

RHEUMATISM–

SEEDS FROM SUNFLOWER PLANT MUST BE EATEN REGULARLY.

DRINK MANGO JUICE AND CHERRY JUICE.

TALK TO YOUR DOCTOR ABOUT MANGANESE SUPPLEMENT.

REMEMBER OVERDOSE OF SOME SUPPLEMENTS CAN BE TOXIC!

S

SCARS

SINUS INFECTIONS

SKIN DISORDERS

STOMACH ULCERS

STREP THROAT

STROKE

SUNBURN

SCARS–

To PREVENT SCARS

VITAMIN E SHOULD BE APPLIED TOPICALLY.

USE MARIGOLD JUICE ON CUTS AND SCRAPES.

SINUS INFECTIONS–

IF YOU HAVE REPEATED SINUS INFECTIONS YOU MAY WANT TO TRY

STONE ROOT/ HERB.

REMEMBER, AIRBORNE ALLERGENS AS WELL AS

ENVIRONMENTAL FACTORS

CAN AFFECT YOUR SINUS PROBLEMS.

EXAMINE YOUR BODY'S RESPONSE

WHEN ELIMINATING PARTICULAR FOODS FROM YOUR DIET.

START WITH COMMON ALLERGENS SUCH AS:

EGGS, WHEAT, PEANUTS,

AND DIARY PRODUCTS.

YOU MAY FIND THAT SOME FOODS ARE THE TROUBLE MAKERS

AND

PETROCHEMICALS WE ALL COMMONLY USE EVERY DAY.

BY ELIMINATING THEM

YOU CAN HELP YOURSELF SIGNIFICANTLY.

SKIN–

For SMOOTHER SKIN

SUNFLOWER SEED (FRESH) MUST BE EATEN.

COD-LIVER OIL SUPPLEMENTS FOR HARD,

DRY OR INFLAMED SKIN MUST BE TAKEN ORALLY.

FISH LIVER OILS MAY PREVENT MANY SKIN DISEASES

SUCH AS ECZEMA.

EAT THE FRUIT POMEGRANATE,

OLD MEDITERRANEAN REMEDY SAYS

IS GOOD FOR YOUR SKIN.

ALSO THE JUICE FROM THE PLANT ALOE VERA

IS VERY GOOD TO YOUR SKIN. FOR YOUNGER LOOKING SKIN

APPLY THE JUICE TOPICALLY. SAYS AN OLD REMEDY.

SKIN THAT IS ROUGH ON THE ELBOWS,

ABOVE THE KNEES AND UPPER ARMS

IS THE SIGN OF VITAMIN A DEFICIENCY.

PERHAPS YOU ARE TAKING VITAMIN A SUPPLEMENT BUT,

DID YOU KNOW, THAT IF YOUR LIVER IS NOT WORKING PROPERLY

YOUR BODY MAY NOT BE ABLE TO USE VITAMIN A?

SKIN CONT.

To MOISTURIZE YOUR SKIN

USE COMBINATION OF OLIVE OIL AND YOUR FAVORITE BODY

WASH.

POUR INTO AN EMPTY BOTTLE—OLIVE OIL (FILL HALF OF THE BOTTLE)

AND THEN ADD BODY WASH IN THE SAME PROPORTION.

SHAKE WELL AND USE IN THE SHOWER TO WASH YOUR BODY WITH IT

AND RINSE.

*

THE ONLY PROBLEM WITH IT IS,

THAT YOU MAY HAVE TO CLEAN YOUR SHOWER MORE OFTEN,

THE OIL WILL STAY ON THE FLOOR, UNLESS YOU WASH IT RIGHT AWAY.

SLEEP–

TROUBLE SLEEPING?

HERE I HAVE SOME SUGGESTIONS:

PUT YOUR BED IN THE MIDDLE OF THE ROOM.

AT LEAST 1 METER FROM EACH WALL,

MAKE SURE YOUR HEAD IS IN THE SOUTH

AND YOUR FEET IN THE NORTH.

A CUP OF WARM MILK WITH A TEA SPOON OF HONEY

RIGHT BEFORE YOU GO TO SLEEP

PROVED TO BE HELPFUL TO SOME.

IF YOU CAN'T SLEEP BECAUSE OF STRESS,

HERE ARE SOME STRESS FORMULAS:

KAVA KAVA, VALERIAN, ST. JOHN'S WORT,

CHAMOMILE TEA, LICORICE TEA

AND LAVENDER TEA.

STOMACH ULCERS–

IF YOU HAVE STOMACH ULCERS DRINK LICORICE TEA.

GET SUPPLEMENT FROM SEAWEED CALLED BLADDERWRACK.

TO PREVENT STOMACH ULCERS

AVOID FERMENTED, PICKLED AND SMOKED FOODS AND

INTRODUCE THE GRAIN AMARANTH TO YOUR DIET.

STREP THROAT–

Much more effective

to rinsing your throat with salty water,

is rinsing with the water solution of herb golden seal.

sage is also good for rinsing

(you can actually mix the two in equal

proportions and have very good rinse).

*

and for fever use:

feverfew/herb or white willow bark /herb.

and bed rest.

don't forget, drink plenty of liquids!

STROKE–

TO PREVENT STROKE TAKE

HAWTHORN BERRIES HERB AND

GINKGO BILOBA HERB SUPPLEMENTS.

*

EAT FRUITS AND VEGETABLES RICH IN VITAMIN C.

SUNBURN–

APPLY OLIVE OIL ON AFFECTED AREA ON DAY FIRST.

YOU MAY HAVE TO REPEAT IT ON THE SECOND DAY.

WATCH YOUR SKIN, IF REDNESS DISAPPEARS

TAKE BATH (DO NOT USE HOT WATER !) AND

GENTLY WITH WASH CLOTH

CLEAN AFFECTED AREA (ONLY WITH WATER). AFTER SKIN DRIES

APPLY OLIVE OIL TO AFFECTED AREA

REPEAT NEXT DAY IF DESIRED.

*

WEAR HATS AND

WEAR PROTECTIVE CLOTHES!

APPLY HIGH SUN PROTECTION PRODUCTS / SUN BLOCK.

T

TEETH

TEETH–

LOOSE TEETH?

DID YOU TRY VITAMIN C FOR IT?

IN GROWING CHILDREN WHILE TEETH ARE BEING FORMED

COD LIVER OIL IS VERY BENEFICIAL.

FOR DENTAL TROUBLES EAT BONE MEAL

(SUPPLEMENT OF CALCIUM AND PHOSPHORUS).

IF YOU HAVE TOOTHACHE-

TRY TO MASSAGE THE GUMS AND TEETH WITH GARLIC.

(MAKE SURE THE JUICE GETS ON THE GUM AND TOOTH).

U

URINARY TRACK INFECTIONS

URINARY TRACK INFECTIONS–

ONE BIG ROOT OF PARSLEY WASH

AND PUT INTO A QUART OF WATER,

BOIL.

LET IT STAND FOR 15-20 MINUTES,

COOL IT DOWN AND DRINK THE LIQUID 3 TIMES A DAY.

DRINK PINEAPPLE AND CRANBERRY JUICE DAILY.

TRY SITTING BATHS—

TO YOUR BATH WATER

ADD APPROXIMATELY 3 TBS. OF SALT.

*

TROUBLE URINATING:

EAT CELERY, DILL AND DRINK LOT'S OF CORNSILK TEA.

V

VARICOSE VEINS

VOMITING / UPSET STOMACH

VARICOSE VEINS–

To GET RID OF VARICOSE VEINS

TAKE SUPPLEMENTS OF HERB CALLED STONE ROOT.

VOMITING / UPSET STOMACH–

Eat plain white toast

DRINK GINGER ALE OR OTHER CLEAR SODA.

W

WARTS

WARTS–

GENTLY MASSAGE IN AFFECTED AREA

JUICE FROM PLANT OF THE NAME

CHELIDONIUM MAJUS.

X

X-RAY

AND OTHER RADIOACTIVE RAYS.

X-RAY

AND OTHER RADIOACTIVE RAYS–

VITAMIN P HAS BEEN USEFUL IN PROTECTING AGAINST

THE HARMFUL EFFECTS OF X-RAY AND OTHER RADIOACTIVE RAYS.

FOODS IN WHICH VITAMIN P IS PRESENT:

GRAPES,

PRUNES,

PLUMS,

BLACK CURRANTS,

ROSE HIPS,

GREEN PEPPERS

AND CITRUS FRUIT (IT IS IN THE WHITE SEGMENTS OF THE FRUIT,

SO DON'T JUICE, EAT THE WHOLE FRUIT!).

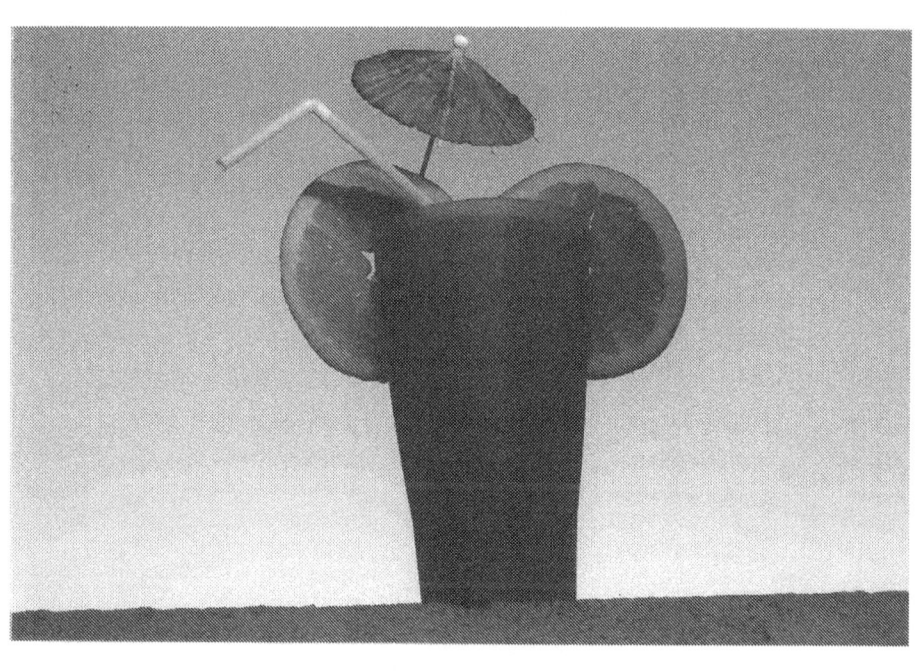

DEAR READER,

IF YOU SUFFER FROM SERIOUS ILLNESS

NEVER ATTEMPT TO HEAL YOURSELF

WITH VITAMINS, MINERALS OR HERBS ON YOUR OWN.

IF YOU HAVE CANCER SOME OF THE METHODS

USED TO TREAT CANCER

DON'T WORK GOOD WITH THE NATURAL REMEDIES

AND CAN BE COUNTER PRODUCTIVE.

-TALK TO YOUR DOCTOR.

*

HERBS USUALLY WORK VERY SLOW,

SO YOU NEED TO BE PATIENT WITH THEM.

NOT EVERY REMEDY WILL WORK FOR EVERYONE IN THE SAME WAY.

HERBS ARE PLANTS WITH POWERFUL HEALING FORCE,

SO USE THEM WISELY . . . .

VITAMINS AND MINERALS ARE VERY IMPORTANT.

IF WE LACK SOME OF THEM WE SUFFER IN MANY DIFFERENT WAYS.

THE KEY IS BALANCE.

*

ALSO LET'S REMEMBER,

OUR LIFE STYLE IS VERY IMPORTANT AND

OUR DIET.

*

KEEP IN MIND THAT OUR ATTITUDE

TOWARD ANOTHER HUMAN BEING IS MORE IMPORTANT

THAN WE OFTEN THINK.

WE NEED MORE LOVE

AND CARE TOWARD ONE ANOTHER

THAN WE HAVE TODAY.

PERHAPS FOR YOUR NEIGHBOR NEXT DOOR

YOU ARE THE ONLY PERSON, WHO MAKES THE DAY SHINE.

GOD BLESS YOU.

L.W.